Improve Digestion *with*

FOOD COMBINING

Steve Meyerowitz

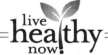

HEALTHY LIVING PUBLICATIONS
Summertown, Tennessee

Cover and interior design: Scattaregia Design

Healthy Living Publications,
a division of Book Publishing Company
P.O. Box 99
Summertown, TN 38483
888-260-8458
bookpubco.com

ISBN 978-1-57067-318-4

20 19 18 17 16 15 14   1 2 3 4 5 6 7 8 9

Library of Congress Cataloging-in-Publication Data

Meyerowitz, Steve.
Improve digestion with food combining / Steve Meyerowitz.
    pages cm
ISBN 978-1-57067-318-4 (pbk.) -- ISBN 978-1-57067-881-3 (e-book)
1. Food combining. 2. Digestion. I. Title.
RA784.M4832 2014
612.3--dc23
                            2014033439

Printed on recycled paper

Book Publishing Company is a member of Green Press Initiative. We chose to print this title on paper with 100% post-consumer recycled content, processed without chlorine, which saved the following natural resources:

- 18 trees
- 563 pounds of solid waste
- 8,414 gallons of water
- 1,551 pounds of greenhouse gases
- 8 million BTU of energy

For more information on Green Press Initiative, visit www.greenpressinitiative.org. Environmental impact estimates were made using the Environmental Defense Fund Paper Calculator. For more information, visit papercalculator.org.

CONTENTS

Introduction

Digestion is not just getting food in and waste out. It's much more than that. In fact, it's the process that nourishes the whole body, governing the absorption and assimilation of nutrients from food. The bottom line: Digestion is responsible for the construction and repair of all the cells in the body.

When you consider food from this angle, isn't it worth examining your approach to eating and how it affects digestion? In one respect, this book plays the very pedestrian role of simply teaching proper eating habits. This involves not only what, where, when, why, and how we eat, but also the consciousness we bring to the essential activity of nourishing ourselves.

Food combining is the process of orchestrating our meals in such a way as to keep the stomach and the rest of the digestive tract sound and happy. Unfortunately, gas, indigestion, distention, sour stomach, and acid reflux are all too common. We know this because the drugs that quell these complaints are the best-selling over-the-counter medicines. All of these symptoms are red flags.

Instead of turning to drugs, we can offset and even prevent such digestive woes with skillful food combining. Knowing which foods are difficult to digest, learning not to overdo it, and recognizing our own habits and limits become even more important as we age. These and other considerations are addressed in the discussion of the five laws of food combining that follow.

If food combining were simply a science governed by the laws of chemistry—and if good digestion were purely the result of formulaic chemical combinations—we could efficiently solve digestive problems by following a food-combining chart. While science and chemistry are valid considerations, other significant factors are at play in achieving optimal digestion: lifestyle, emotions, attitude, timing, habits, and environment all contribute to the "art" of food combining. Together, the science and art of food combining affect much of our daily lives, figuring into the soundness of our stomachs and our health overall.

The good news is that we can change our lives simply by cultivating good eating habits and shunning bad ones. Relearning our relationship to food—what we eat and how we eat it—has a ripple effect not only on health but also on lifestyle. My advice is to eat consciously, judiciously, and apply common sense. Most of all, enjoy your food and be happy. Then you'll digest every bite.

The Laws of Food Combining

It's not a crime to have poor eating habits, but that doesn't mean you won't be punished for them. In the short run, there's stomachache, headache, indigestion, flatulence, and diarrhea. Many people routinely experience uncomfortable symptoms like these—sometimes for years—and pay no attention to them. Over time, however, failings in the digestive process give way to acute and chronic diseases, including arthritis, colon cancer, eczema, fibromyalgia, hypoglycemia, irritable bowel syndrome, and ulcers.

Your digestion need not be subject to such difficulties, though. Bring order to your eating and take control of your health by following the five laws of food combining. Rein in quantity and regularity. Approach eating consciously and rethink the order in which you consume certain foods. And reschool yourself in the chemical properties of foods, such as proteins, starches, sugars, and fats. Whether you've been diagnosed with an ulcer at age fifty or are trying to eliminate food sensitivities in your five-year-old grandchild, you can take the five laws into your own hands.

Law I: Quantity

Quantity is the first law of digestion. Overconsumption is the number one cause of indigestion. Our appetites are far ahead of our stomachs. We can go a long way toward better digestion—and better health—by remembering that we can only handle so much. If we want optimal digestion and superior health, we must practice self-control and make a conscious decision to monitor food intake at every meal.

One way to keep track of your eating habits is to write them down in a diary. Note established patterns. You may find yourself repeatedly seduced into self-destructive habits. Perhaps you have a voracious appetite and consume food in desperation. Ask yourself, why? Were you deprived of food as a child? Or were you trained to finish everything on your plate, even if you were full? Now that your circumstances have changed, isn't it time to kick these habits?

Sometimes food can be used as a substitute for love. Many folks who feel or have felt unloved compensate for this lack by overeating. They succumb to a variety of tantalizing and sumptuous dishes that reward them with the pleasure that makes up for lost love—at least temporarily. This and other harmful strategies are sure to backfire.

If overeating is a problem for you, try to become conscious of what you're eating and take smaller portions. In addition, pay attention to *how* you're eating, which can affect the quantity of food you consume. For example, do you stuff your mouth with far more than you can chew? Incomplete chewing results in premature swallowing, which initiates a chain reaction of problems. Perhaps you chew and talk at the same time, allowing air to enter the stomach and increasing the likelihood that you'll swallow incompletely chewed food. Or maybe you are a speed eater or guzzle down lots of water with every gulp. These bad habits, in combination with overeating, are a sure recipe for poor digestion.

Law 2: Regularity

Regularity, the second law of digestion, pertains to how you fit eating into your daily schedule and the variety of foods you eat. Yes, the timing of your meals counts. Maybe you're so busy, you put off eating until you're absolutely famished. People who don't eat during the day often end up gorging themselves at night. Food eaten late at night is poorly digested because the organs of digestion are in a resting and cleansing phase. Also, the secretion of digestive enzymes is reduced when you're lying down. The result is that food sits in the stomach and isn't digested properly, and sleep is often disturbed.

On the other hand, what if you eat too much throughout the day? Perhaps you're a full-time homemaker, always near the kitchen and tempted to nosh all the time. The biggest curse of an ad hoc eater may be the loss of digestive power. At any given time, the supply of digestive enzymes is limited. After a meal, this supply is exhausted. Sufficient time must elapse so the stomach can generate new digestive juices and the digestive system can rest. When heavy foods or meals are eaten in succession, the system is overloaded and normal digestion becomes impossible. The result is a digestive tract that breeds disease. Instead of an efficient machine, you have a traffic jam. And food that stays in the intestines too long, or that travels through too slowly, ferments and putrefies, affecting overall health and well-being.

While there are many incorrect approaches to regularity, it's fairly easy to get it right, sometimes without trying. Some people unintentionally benefit from an imposed meal schedule because of the logistics of their daily lives. Their mealtimes may be fixed to conform with their work schedules or those of family members. This is fortunate, because the ideal way to eat is to be as regular in your habits as possible, both in terms of the timing of meals and the variety of foods eaten. If you have breakfast at eight o'clock, lunch at one, and dinner at six every day, your digestive system will function better than that of someone whose mealtimes are unstructured.

The effect of an external schedule has an internal, physiological benefit. Your juices start to flow at dinner time and you become hungry. The ideal schedule features meals that are five or six hours apart. Small snacks of fruits or liquids in between meals will not usually interfere with the digestive process.

Routine consumption of the same foods is also a key to regularity. Frequently switching up the content of your meals forces your digestive organs to constantly readapt to new foods. Ideally, a diet should be designed in concentric circles, with a group of primary foods (eaten every week) in the center and secondary or accessory foods (garlic, onions, olive oil, salt, and condiments) in an outer ring. In a ring around these foods is another group that may be chosen once or twice per month. For example, perhaps you include mushrooms or avocados in your diet, but only on an every-other-week basis. Beyond this group lies a culinary twilight zone, where unusual and exotic foods (or, at least, unusual to you) are enjoyed only on special occasions, such as when you're dining out, attending a wedding, or traveling. For example, you may never include artichoke hearts, Brussels sprouts, or kiwifruit on your shopping list, but you savor these foods during holidays or occasional events.

This doesn't mean you should never eat foods that aren't at the core of your diet; however, indulging in unusual foods may result in some digestive rumblings. Radical shifts in diet can disrupt your whole system and lead to sleeplessness, irritability, headaches, fatigue, gas, heartburn, and even colds. On the other hand, being regular in your diet, both in terms of timing and mainstay foods, creates regularity—an efficiently working digestion machine.

Law 3: Conscious Eating

Conscious eating, the third law of digestion, requires that we know what to eat, when to eat, and when to stop. The most digestive energy is available to us if we eat when we're genuinely hungry. For example, when a farmer has worked many hours in the field, he arrives at the dinner table with a robust appetite. He's physically hungry. His body has burned a lot of calories and, after a brief (but important) rest, he's ready to dig in to a well-deserved meal. You can be sure his food will be thoroughly digested. His digestive system is primed to receive and process it. On the other hand, someone who is not really hungry and eats, for example, because the group is eating, brings little systemic preparedness and digestive strength to his meal. The result is likely to be some form of indigestion.

No one can teach you to determine when you're hungry. Hunger is part of your instinctual mechanism. You either experience it or you don't. The problem in modern civilized societies is that the average person never experiences true hunger. Food is always around. But, if you pay attention to your sense of hunger and abide by it, your ability to digest and assimilate nutrients will increase significantly. In addition to eating only when you're hungry, stop eating when your stomach feels half full (the mind is slower to recognize fullness than the stomach). Don't be discouraged if you're unable to identify this halfway point at first. Your ability will improve with each meal.

A major cause of overeating is the inelegant habit of overfilling the mouth. Fill your mouth too full and you'll force food down your gullet before it's sufficiently chewed, causing—at the very least—mild indigestion and gas. To avoid such unpleasant results, take in small amounts with each bite and don't add more until the last bite is fully chewed.

Another aspect of eating consciously is pacing yourself and not eating too quickly. Chew more slowly. Make a deliberate attempt to stretch out your meal and avoid eating when you're in a rush. Food eaten too quickly is not sufficiently broken down, resulting in flatulence, distension, poor absorption, vitamin deficiencies, irritable colon, and nervous stomach—not to mention laying the groundwork for more complex problems. The aim is to masticate the food into a bolus (a fluid mass) before swallowing. Chew your food into the tiniest pieces possible. This creates more surface area on which stomach acid can act. The simple, mechanical act of mastication can make a world of difference to digestion and to the assimilation of nutrients.

One of the best ways to counter unconscious eating is to take a moment to appreciate your meal before you begin. Almost all religions have some form of pre-meal ritual—a prayer or a thanksgiving—but this pause for reflection need not be religious at all. Everyone benefits by spending a few moments before a meal to quiet the mind and relax the body. You may thank the earth for bringing forth her nourishing foods or thank the people who took part in their preparation. Or you may thank the universe for allowing you at this time and place to nourish your body while others, less fortunate, cannot. The goal is to take a small amount of time to focus on the act of eating and relax the body. Take a deep breath, count to twenty-five, then begin your meal.

Some religious practices call for silence with each meal. This relaxes the whole body and is ideal for focusing on the stomach and the act of eating. Silence affords the ultimate in food consciousness. You're calm and your thoughts are free to settle on the food and the feelings that it inspires in you. And there's another, very practical reason not to talk while eating: talk while you eat and you'll swallow air right along with your food, creating burping and sometimes hiccups.

If silence is not possible, keep the conversation calm and light. In too many households, mealtimes do double duty, serving as a time to eat and a forum for family business, gossip, and the release of anger and frustrations. The dinner table becomes a boxing ring in which family arguments play out. This is how heartburn, reflux, ulcers, and other digestive problems start.

The table should not be a combat zone. Instead, it should provide your ideal eating environment. How do candlelight, white dinner napkins, china, and Mozart sound? Whether or not this is your style, such a setting is wonderful for digestion. Soft music goes great with a meal, as does a peaceful ambiance. Even the family picnic can promote good digestion if the atmosphere is relaxed, with plenty of fresh air and good cheer.

And finally, observe all aspects of your meal. When you sit down to eat, invite all your senses to join in. Take time to bring your awareness to how your food smells, looks, and tastes. Pass on anything that doesn't seem quite right to you. Honor important cues that may indicate that a particular food is not a good choice at a particular time.

Law 4: Sequence

The order in which you introduce different foods into your system during the course of a meal or a series of meals is important. This sequence contributes enormously to successful digestion, absorption, and assimilation. This is the fourth law of digestion. There are different theories on how to organize a meal, and opinions about the proper order in which to eat various foods are, to say the least, likely to spur disagreement. However, you'll be rewarded if you make a sensible effort to arrange your meal so that foods flow harmoniously through your digestive tract. A well-ordered meal permits your stomach to function smoothly, resulting in shorter digestion times and better assimilation of nutrients. This means less gas, bloating, heartburn, and similar symptoms and a happier, more energetic feeling after the meal is over.

One theory is that foods that are easy to digest should be consumed before more complex foods (see box, page 13). Trouble starts when various types of foods, such as those that digest at different rates and require different digestive enzymes, clash with foods from other groups.

Foods can be categorized according to such attributes as density, water content, and complexity of fats, carbohydrates, and proteins. The denser and more complex a food, the longer its journey through the digestive tract and the greater the delay before absorption and assimilation. Mixing foods of different categories and densities complicates digestion and slows the whole system.

Water, Juices, and Other Thin Liquids

The easiest foods to digest are liquids: fruit and vegetable juices, light vegetable broths, most soups, and so on. The easiest of these are juices, such as apple, carrot, celery, and spinach juice. Because they spend no appreciable time in the stomach, juices can be enjoyed even by those with weak digestion. In fact, juices go right into the intestines, and more than 95 percent of their nutrients are absorbed into the bloodstream and assimilated into your cells. If you're not digesting your food well, get your vitamins instead from fresh fruit and vegetable juices. Herbal teas are also nutritive and healing, as are vegetable broths. Broths can be homemade or purchased in powdered form, and they're very nourishing and easy to digest.

Sensible Order of Ingestion

Give some thought to the sequence of the foods you consume, and your digestive system will thank you. This order is most likely to create harmony:

1. water, juices, and other thin liquids
2. non-starchy fruit, smoothies (blended foods), and soups
3. vegetables
4. beans and grains
5. other high-protein foods

Here is how sequencing might work during mealtimes:

Breakfast

1. juice
2. fruit
3. cereal

Lunch

1. drink
2. fruit, vegetable, or salad
3. sandwich (grains with beans or other high-protein food)

Dinner

1. drink
2. salad
3. main dish (grains, beans, or other high-protein food)
   with vegetable

Fresh, Non-starchy Fruits

Fruits are next up on the list of easy-to-digest foods. Non-starchy fruits have the most water of all the solid foods. In fact, their water content can be as high as 90 percent. Aptly named, the watermelon is a prime example. After juicing a huge slice, you're left with only a few tablespoons of pulp. Most of the fruit is water. On the other extreme, a banana yields no water—it's all pulp. Bananas are a starchy fruit and unusual as fruits go.

Other non-starchy fruits, such as apples, berries, cherries, citrus, melons, peaches, pears, and plums, are easily digested and generally spend between thirty and sixty minutes in the stomach. Since they contain mostly water and soft fiber, no heavy protein- or starch-digesting enzymes or strong acids are required.

It's a different story with some other fruits, however. Bananas, avocados, and coconuts are high in fat, protein, or carbohydrates and take longer to digest. Dried fruits, such as raisins, figs, and dates, are high in fiber and sugar. They contain only about 10 percent water, so they differ enormously from non-starchy fruits. They also spend more time in the stomach—generally forty-five minutes to an hour and a half, depending on quantity. Fatty fruits and dried fruits are in a league of their own and don't accurately reflect the common attributes of fruits. They belong lower down on the list of digestible foods because they're more complex.

Smoothies and Blended Foods

Be aware that not everything you can drink is easy to digest. For example, if you blend bananas and apple juice, you aren't making banana-apple juice. Rather, you're making a smoothie, a purée of bananas. Drink a smoothie, and you're really eating solid food, only the blender has "chewed" it for you instead of your teeth! This is the difference between blending and juicing. A blender purées or liquefies a solid food. A juicer extracts the water content from a fruit or vegetable and separates it from the pulp. The higher the solid content of a liquid, the harder it is to digest.

One popular substitute for dairy milk is almond milk, which is easy to make. Just process almonds with water or apple juice in a blender and then strain. If you don't strain the almond milk, you'll be drinking solid bits of almond. If you have weak digestion, nut milk is an excellent choice, but make sure you strain out as many of the solids as possible.

Also, be aware that the solids of some foods, such as cashews, bananas, and papayas, can't be removed by straining. If you blend cashews to make cashew milk (which is delicious, by the way) and pour it through a strainer, the entire contents will pass through, leaving nothing behind. Similarly, when bananas and mangoes are run through a juicer, no pulp is left behind. When you juice or strain these foods, the end result will be a solid. Please enjoy them. They are wonderful. But don't be fooled into thinking that cashew milk is easier to digest than cashews and don't assume that there is such a thing as mango or papaya juice just because you see bottled versions in a store. Read the ingredients and you'll find that such "juices" are really purées of these fruits thinned with the juice from apples, grapes, or other fruits.

Soups

Soups are the most difficult to categorize because there are so many different kinds. For example, there's a vast difference between a vegetable broth and a hearty bean soup. Beans are hard to digest, and despite the fact that it's semifluid, a thick lentil soup is as difficult to digest as a plate of lentils.

When it comes to digestibility, each soup has to be looked at individually. Some may challenge digestion because they contain high-protein ingredients. Or they may include additives, such as MSG, artificial flavors, or thickeners. For example, flour may be added to thicken a soup, so if you're allergic to wheat, you would have difficulty digesting that soup.

The easiest soup to digest is a light vegetable soup or broth. To make one, just chop up some vegetables—such as asparagus, broccoli, or spinach—add spices, then add water, and simmer. Strain out the vegetables and drink the broth, which is easy to digest and super nutritious. Like juices and water, broths are best taken at the beginning of a meal.

Vegetables

Green leafy vegetables have almost as much water as fruits, making them quick and easy to digest. Some other vegetables, such as tomatoes and cucumbers, also can be digested as quickly as fruits. In fact, botanists define tomatoes and cucumbers as fruits because they contain seeds, although these foods are commonly identified as vegetables. A simple salad featuring these ingredients can take as little as one hour to pass through your stomach.

Of course, we also have to take the dressing into consideration. The type of salad dressing and how much you use can complicate the digestibility of a salad. A dressing made with pure olive oil and lemon juice, for example, will minimally extend the digestion time of a salad because the oil will coat the greens, making them slightly harder to digest. However, a dressing made with nut or seed butters (such as tahini) will take even longer, as will dairy-based dressings, such as ranch or blue cheese. Of course, fancy salads, such as those that contain fruit, cheese, nuts, or croutons, are even harder to digest because they mix different food groups and include high-fat and high-protein ingredients. These salads, or a salad that includes grains (such as tabouli with bulgur), will be more difficult to digest than a simple green salad.

Green leafy vegetables can be digested more quickly than starchy vegetables. Asparagus, broccoli, Brussels sprouts, cauliflower, and summer squash, for example, are so starchy, they're usually eaten cooked. Steaming a starchy vegetable, such as broccoli, softens the fiber, breaks down the starch, and adds water to the vegetable, making it easier to digest.

Some vegetables can be eaten either raw or cooked. Cabbage is frequently served raw in salads and coleslaw. It has a lot of fiber. However, raw cabbage can cause gas for many people, making steamed cabbage an easier-to-digest alternative. All members of the cabbage family—which also includes broccoli, bok choy, collard greens, kale, and Swiss chard—can be gently steamed for better digestibility, especially if eaten in quantity. Other common vegetables, such as carrots and beets, are more fibrous than starchy. They're very high in water content and very juicy, but their fiber can keep you chewing for a long time. Because of the fiber, these vegetables also take longer to digest than green leafy vegetables.

Potatoes, other tubers, and squashes are the starchiest members of the vegetable family and, when eaten after baking, take approximately two hours to pass through your stomach. This group includes sweet potatoes, yams, red potatoes, russet potatoes, rutabagas, and acorn and butternut squash. Preparation methods other than baking can enhance digestibility. For example, steamed potatoes are easier to digest than baked potatoes because they're softened by the cooking water. Some people prefer baked potatoes, however, because more nutrients are retained.

Some more exotic members of the vegetable family are mushrooms, sea vegetables, and sprouts. Mushrooms are high in protein and are considered the "meat" of the vegetable kingdom. One and a half hours is the average digestion time for shiitake, oyster, and other common edible mushrooms. Sea vegetables, such as dulse, kelp, and nori, are grown in the ocean and are comparable to green leafy vegetables in terms of digestion. Green leafy sprouts, such as alfalfa, buckwheat, clover, radish, sunflower, and other leafy (but not bean) sprouts, are also classed in the same family as green leafy vegetables. Because they're so young and have such tender fiber, sprouts are more comparable to fruits than vegetables. Allow less than an hour for a meal of green leafy sprouts to digest. Generally, nothing in the vegetable kingdom, if eaten in moderation, takes longer than two hours to digest.

Beans and Grains

In terms of digestibility, beans and grains are next in line after starchy vegetables. Both are composed predominantly of starch, are considered respectable protein foods, and even have a fair amount of essential oils. In general, beans and grains can take between two and a half to three and a half hours to digest, depending on the quantity consumed.

Glutinous grains, such as wheat, spelt, Kamut, rye, and barley, cause digestive troubles for those who are sensitive to gluten. Gluten is the white, sticky protein that's responsible for holding bread together. Whole grains are slightly easier to digest than products made from those grains, such as breads, cookies, and crackers. This is partly because the bread-making and manufacturing processes make the gluten more viscous and sticky. Non-glutinous grains, such as amaranth, buckwheat (kasha), corn, millet, rice, and quinoa, are generally easier to digest than glutinous grains. Of these, millet and buckwheat are the lightest and least concentrated grains, and therefore are digested more quickly than the others. Corn causes some allergies and is fairly tough to digest. Amaranth and quinoa are the highest in protein of all grains but still fairly easy to digest.

Sprouted wheat (wheat is the most practical grain for sprouting) is easier to digest than unsprouted wheat and contains less gluten. Sprouting transforms the starch in the grain, making raw sprouted wheat edible, albeit only in small quantities. Soft wheat, commonly used in pastries, has less gluten and less protein and is easier to digest than common bread wheat. Sprouted soft wheat is pre-digested enough to eat as a raw snack. However, because sprouted grains are still raw, they cannot be consumed in the same voluminous quantity as cooked grains.

On average, beans (legumes) take longer to digest than grains. Generally, beans have about 10 percent more protein. Soybeans can have as much as 40 percent protein, whereas amaranth, quinoa, and wheat have only 20 percent. This gives beans their reputation as respectable sources of protein, but they're still mostly starch.

When picked fresh or sprouted, peas can be eaten raw and are among the easiest beans to digest. Lentils, mung beans, and adzuki beans can also be eaten raw after sprouting. Some beans, however, such as chickpeas (garbanzo beans) and soybeans, are difficult to digest raw, even after sprouting. When beans are sprouted, cooking time is decreased because sprouting breaks down starch and protein.

Tofu and tempeh are two popular soybean-based foods. Tofu is made from curdled soy milk. It's very light and versatile. If you have trouble digesting soy, this may be the one soy food you can consume. However, if you're allergic to soy, it would still be a verboten food. Expect tofu, by itself, to digest in under two hours. Tempeh is a fermented, bacteria-cultured food. Even though fermentation pre-digests the beans, tempeh is still considered a concentrated food and takes two and a half to three and a half hours to digest.

Nuts and Seeds

As a category, nuts and seeds take longer to digest than grains and beans, although, of course, it depends on the quantity consumed. They're definitely more complex: some nuts are 45 percent total fat, 25 percent protein, 20 percent carbohydrates, and less than 10 percent water. As a group, nuts and seeds have more protein and fat (the two most difficult components to digest) than grains and beans. Just rub a few pecans or Brazil nuts in your hand to feel their oil. It soon becomes obvious that these concentrated foods must be consumed judiciously and in moderation.

The digestion of nuts and seeds would not be a problem if it were not for commercial processing. In their natural state, all nuts and seeds come with a protective covering—shells. These hard shells are almost impossible to remove without the aid of nutcrackers. From a digestion standpoint, the shells are signposts warning "eater beware." Modern shelling machines efficiently remove the shells from nuts and seeds, such as almonds, Brazil nuts, peanuts, sunflower seeds, walnuts, and others. The problem is that the convenience of shelled nuts and seeds seduces us into eating them quickly and in greater quantities. If they had not been artificially liberated by machines, the handful of almonds that we now wolf down in two minutes would likely take fifteen minutes to eat if we had to do the shelling. That extra amount of time enhances good digestion because it establishes a gradual pace of consumption and naturally prevents overeating.

The most difficult nuts to digest are the ones that contain the highest percentages of oil, such as Brazil nuts, macadamia nuts, pecans, pine nuts, and walnuts. Macadamia nuts, which come from Hawaii and Australia, win the prize for the nut with the highest fat content—a whopping 76 percent.

Such high oil content raises another problem—rancidity. Once nuts are shelled, they lose their natural protection from the elements and deteriorate upon exposure to heat, light, and air. When possible, eat nuts that you shell yourself. They're freshest that way, and again, shelling them by hand discourages overconsumption.

Nut butters, such as almond butter, cashew butter, sunflower butter, tahini, and, of course, the ubiquitous peanut butter, combine thousands of nuts or seeds in one jar, making a super-concentrate of an already complex food that is packed with oil, protein, and carbohydrates. When nuts or nut butters are prominent in a full-sized meal, it will take two to three hours for your stomach to empty.

Despite these hard facts, don't shun nuts and seeds and their butters. They're wonderful sources of protein, essential oils, and minerals. Just eat them prudently.

Other High-Protein Foods

Dairy products are even more complex than nuts and seeds. In addition to protein, they contain carbohydrates and fat. The more you mix proteins, carbohydrates, and fats, all prominent in animal-based foods, the more complex the meal becomes. For the best results, pair high-protein foods with vegetables only and avoid starches and other types of protein. Multiple proteins increase the strain on your digestive abilities; if you mix too many, you're likely to lose vigor and experience fatigue, flatulence, and putrefaction.

Deep-Fried Foods

Foods prepared by deep-frying in oils are by far the most difficult to digest as well as the most unhealthy. Stir-frying is better because the oil doesn't impregnate the food as much as it does in deep-frying. Deep-frying oil is so denatured that it's beyond the point of digestibility! Oils in commercial and fast-food restaurant fryers are used over and over all day long. Not only are these degraded oils harder to digest, they are dangerous. Their molecular structure collapses and forms dangerous substances, such as aldehydes, acrylamides, and peroxides—all carcinogens.

Putting It All Together

The ideal meal in terms of digestion is made up of one food or one family of foods. Digestion of a simple meal is quick, easy, and efficient. For example, a meal that mixes oranges with grapefruits would be easy to digest because both foods are from the same family (fruit) and the same class (citrus). The same thing can be said for apples and pears. Because these fruits are so similar, the stomach recognizes them as the same food. This is also the case for other food combos, including peaches and plums, cantaloupe and honeydew melon, raisins and currants, and all the berries.

Each food group differs in taste, texture, and nutrition, so naturally each group is treated differently by the digestive system. Combining salad greens is excellent: Bibb lettuce, Boston lettuce, endive, romaine, and green

Consider a Combo

Mixing fruits and vegetables is usually taboo. But there are some exceptions: apples, lemons, and limes pair wonderfully with vegetables. In fact, these fruits make great additions to vegetable juice.

leafy sprouts are all treated as one food as far as digestion goes. The addition of dill, parsley, or spinach is also excellent because they're in the same class—green leafy vegetables. Although mixing one group of vegetables with another results in a *good* combination, using only those of the same class—such as the cabbage family—results in an *excellent* combination. For some other examples of excellent combinations, see the box below.

Care should be taken when pairing nuts with other foods. Consume nuts with salads and non-starchy vegetables. When taken in moderation, nuts also combine well with most fruits. Nuts are frequently served with dried fruits, which help break up their concentration. Don't eat nuts with grains or beans or starches because, as you'll see, they require different types of digestive enzymes.

Easy-to-Digest Combinations

Eat foods within each of these groups for easiest digestibility. Eat 1 through 5 together for good digestion, and 6 through 9 together for good digestion. Number 10 should be eaten alone or together with numbers 3, 4, or 5.

1. all melons
2. all citrus fruits
3. peaches and plums
4. apples and pears
5. all dried fruits
6. all green leafy vegetables
7. all starchy vegetables
8. all beans and peas
9. all bean sprouts
10. all nuts and seeds

Law 5: Chemistry

Everyone thinks that the most important issue in food combining is the chemical makeup of the different foods, the fifth law of digestion. However, for most of us, chemistry is at best a difficult subject, and the effort to juggle foods according to their chemical composition creates too much mental stress for something that is supposed to be a pleasurable activity. Still, it's beneficial to understand the basic building blocks of food.

Protein

Protein has the reputation for being our most important nutrient, but it's overvalued. True, its role in building and repairing cells is indisputable. But our modern preoccupation with protein comes mostly from the mistaken belief that it's required in large quantities and comes only from limited and select sources. Although this is a subject that goes beyond the discussion of food combining, it's worth addressing briefly. There are three misconceptions: (1) we need a minimum number of grams of protein daily based on body weight and age; (2) protein is available only in a limited number of foods; (3) each meal must provide "complete" proteins.

These outmoded concepts were popularized by uninformed doctors and sometimes by nutrition writers. Frances Moore Lappé, in her book *Diet for a Small Planet*, expounded the theory that protein foods had to be carefully combined to supply the body with the right amount of the various protein components, namely amino acids. Not everyone agreed with her at the time, and in the years since, the almost political controversy she initiated ended with a rare event: a retraction! In articles and books she has written since, Lappé has stated that combining protein foods on a meal-by-meal basis is unnecessary.

The most well-known protein foods are animal-based foods (such as chicken and beef), legumes, nuts, and seeds. However, the fact is that every food has protein, since protein is required for all cell growth. But the relative proportions of protein, starch, and sugar determine whether an item is considered a "protein food." Soybeans, for example, with 16.5 percent protein and 10 percent starch, are a protein food. Most beans, however, are predominantly starch. For instance, pinto beans are about 8 percent protein and 25 percent starch. In combination, starches and proteins are difficult to digest, even when nature itself has put them together. That's one reason why beans should be eaten with respect.

You may be surprised to learn that the foods highest in protein are vegetarian. Spirulina and chlorella, two ancient varieties of algae that grow in high-altitude lakes, contain about 60 percent protein. Nutritional yeast (a food manufactured by friendly microorganisms) and barley and wheat grass powder are between 35 and 50 percent protein. Other good vegan protein foods are grains and beans, including wheat and soy foods, and nuts and seeds. For maximum digestibility, it's best to eat one protein food at a time. Proteins can be classified by groups, such as grains. Proteins from beans fall in another category, and these two categories happen to mix well. However, animal-based proteins, such as beef, chicken, and cheese, each require their own special enzyme brew. Including all of these different proteins together in one meal is a prescription for digestive disaster. Too many different protein foods exhaust both you and your digestive juices, leaving you with that dull, sleepy feeling. Worse, putrefaction can develop from undigested proteins. For the chronic abuser, this can mean the beginning of colon, liver, and skin problems and other related chronic conditions.

You might think that acidic foods, such as citrus fruits, would be helpful in digesting protein. On the contrary, fruit acids can limit the production of stomach acid by giving your system mixed signals. When protein enters the mouth, the nerve endings on the tongue alert the stomach glands to secrete hydrochloric acid and pepsin, which are needed to digest protein. But the juices for digesting citrus are not the same as those required for digesting proteins. So even though eggs and orange juice are part of the typical American breakfast, they don't make good companions in the stomach.

Starches

Starches are the most common food elements in most people's diets. Starches belong to the larger family of carbohydrates, which is the predominant food category in nature. Carbohydrates are simply a combination of carbon and water. All plants and grasses are carbohydrates. Also included in this family are sugar and cellulose (indigestible fiber). Starches are our best source of fuel for muscular activity, so if you're a big starch eater and your body doesn't require the fuel, starches will be converted into fat and stored in adipose tissue.

Ironic though it may sound, indigestible starches play an indispensable role in digestion. Cellulose, hemicellulose, lignins, and pectins come from the fibrous portions of foods, including the skins of fruits, the stalks of vegetables, and the hulls of seeds and grains. Although such items are broken by the masticating action of teeth and softened by stomach acid, they're never dissolved. Still, fibrous foods are essential because they provide roughage and facilitate the wavelike motion, known as peristalsis, of food through the intestines.

Squashes, such as acorn, buttercup, and butternut, are excellent starches. So are such vegetables as broccoli, Brussels sprouts, and cauliflower. Beans, including black beans, chickpeas, lentils, and lima beans, are known as respectable protein sources, but they're also starchy. Other starchy foods are grains, such as barley, corn, oats, rice, and wheat, and the foods derived from them. In addition, the starch category includes highly processed foods, such as white bread and instant potatoes, which I don't recommend. There are also starchy junk foods, such as crackers, French fries, potato chips, pretzels, and so forth. Once the vitamins, fibers, and enzymes have been removed, these foods are harder to digest, since our bodies must supply the missing nutrients to facilitate digestion. The only thing that's superior about these processed starches is their shelf life.

The more you chew starchy foods, the better. Chewing increases the surface area for saliva to work on, which is the first step in the digestion of starchy foods. However, this enzymatic action stops if a protein food is eaten at the same time as a starch. If starchy foods are eaten first and enough time is allowed for them to pass through the stomach, then protein foods can be digested without any interference. But if protein and starch foods are combined, starch digestion will be slowed down until the protein food is digested. The starch then exits the stomach in a semi-digested state, sending incompletely digested food into the small intestine.

Just as acidic foods don't aid the digestion of proteins, they can be problematic when it comes to digesting starch. Even one or two teaspoons of vinegar has enough acetic acid to suspend salivary digestion completely. Acidic fruits also can inhibit the digestion of starch. This means tomatoes, berries, grapes, sour apples, and citrus fruits will interfere with starch digestion. There is even some evidence that these foods not only inhibit the digestive enzyme ptyalin, but they're also strong enough to destroy it. So if you like orange juice with your toast in the morning, try drinking it ten minutes before consuming the bread.

Sugar

Sugar is the simplest type of carbohydrate, and the simplest forms of sugar, monosaccharides, include glucose, fructose, and galactose. Honey, milk, and fruit contain monosaccharides. Glucose, also called blood sugar or dextrose, is the only kind of monosaccharide the body uses. The liver converts fructose (fruit sugar) and galactose (milk sugar) to glucose for use by the body.

Two monosaccharides linked together are called disaccharides. The most common disaccharide is sucrose. Sucrose contains glucose and fructose and is the type of sugar in beets, maple syrup, and sugarcane. It's the form of sugar commonly used in commercial foods, from candies to soda pop. Eating too many sucrose-rich foods will drain your energy because they use up B vitamins and minerals. Lactose, a disaccharide in milk, is the hardest sugar of all to digest because it requires the enzyme lactase, which is abundant in children and scarce in adults. Many people experience sensitivities and indigestion when consuming milk products for this reason. Maltose is a disaccharide that is a by-product of the digestion of starch in grains and is also available in the form of barley malt and rice syrup.

Sugar, whether a monosaccharide or disaccharide, is one of the easiest foods to digest. Even water dissolves it. And it spends very little time in the stomach. However, sugar inhibits the secretion of gastric juice. Sugar also inhibits the secretion of the enzyme ptyalin, which is needed to break down starch. Even if you chew well and mechanically break down your bread or pasta, for example, little or no chemical digestion will take place in the stomach. The bread gets to the small intestine before it can be digested. Conversely, the passage of sugar is slowed by the presence of starch. The longer sugar stays in the stomach, the greater the chance fermentation will take place. Fermentation is the breakdown of sugar into alcohol and carbon dioxide. Carbon dioxide causes gas and distension, and alcohol robs the body of B vitamins.

Fermentation results when protein and sugar are eaten together. Again, sugar foods don't need to spend much time in the stomach, so when sugar is consumed alone, it moves along quickly to the small intestine. But protein foods can take hours to make this trip. Therefore, rather than passing right through on its own time schedule, the fruit, candy, or other sugary food has to wait sometimes for a couple of hours while the protein food digests. During this time, the sugar ferments in the warm, moist environment of the stomach. Ordinarily, stomach acid would prevent fermentation, but sugar inhibits the full secretion of gastric juice. (This is why eating sweets before a meal can spoil the appetite.) If the meal is big enough to stimulate a certain amount of gastric secretion, the subsequent release of carbon dioxide will drive stomach acid into the esophagus, giving you that burning feeling known as heartburn.

Fats

Fats are the most difficult of all the nutrients to digest and take the longest to move through the digestive system. But don't avoid fats for this reason. Rather, do your best to keep your overall fat intake in balance with the rest of your diet and select the finest oils and oil-rich whole foods.

Fats play essential roles in human health. They provide more calories (heat energy) than any other food: fats offer 9 calories per gram as compared to 4 calories per gram from proteins and carbohydrates. In addition, fats help cushion the internal organs, line and protect parts of the central nervous system, feed the skin and hair, insulate against heat loss, absorb and transport fat-soluble vitamins, and regulate fat metabolism.

The most important members of the fat family are the polyunsaturates, which include linoleic, arachidonic, and linolenic acids (the omega-3, -6, and -9 acids). They're known as essential fatty acids because they must be ingested (the body doesn't manufacture them) and are necessary for normal cell growth and function. Coconut, hemp, flax, safflower, sesame, soybean, and sunflower oils are excellent sources. Other recommended sources of essential fatty acids (which also happen to be relatively easy to digest) are almonds, olives, pecans, pumpkin seeds, sunflower seeds, walnuts, and wheat germ.

The fat content of a meal determines how slowly food will move through your digestive tract. Fat digestion supersedes protein and carbohydrate digestion, since enzymes must first work on the fat to separate the different nutrients. A big meal with a high fat content can potentially stay in the stomach for three or more hours before it reaches the duodenum, the passageway between the stomach and the small intestine. The nerve endings here send signals to the gallbladder to secrete bile. Bile emulsifies fats and starts the secretion of additional enzymes that further digest and separate the fats from the bile salts. The emulsified fats are now soluble enough to pass through the walls of the small intestine on their way to the liver. The liver combines oils with protein, forming lipoproteins that are distributed to the cells and tissues, resulting in healthy skin and hair.

No discussion of fats is complete without covering solid, or saturated, fats, which are usually associated with animal-based foods, and oils, which are liquids squeezed from grains, nuts, and seeds. As the term "solid fats" implies, some fats remain solid at room temperature. Palm and coconut oils are two vegetable fats that remain solid at room temperature. Animal-based fats are mostly saturated, while vegetable oils are mostly unsaturated. Saturation means that the molecules in the oil have been filled in with hydrogen atoms; in unsaturated fats, the molecules remain open. Unsaturated fats are easier to digest and absorb than saturated fats, so it follows that vegetable oils are easier to digest than animal fats.

Liquid vegetable oils can be made solid through the undesirable process of hydrogenation, which adds hydrogen atoms. The result is margarine, shortening, and peanut butter that doesn't separate. Food manufacturers use hydrogenation to increase shelf life, make products creamy, and discourage rancidity. Unfortunately, vitamins, minerals, and essential fatty acids are destroyed in the hydrogenation process. Worse still, hydrogenated oils are hard to digest, with more effort required to break the molecular bonds.

In the stomach, fat digestion is assisted by acids, enzymes, vitamins, minerals, and phospholipids. Phospholipids, such as lecithin, are a natural ingredient of many oil-rich foods. They help emulsify fats and are found in every cell in the body, especially in the liver, brain, and nervous system. The more unrefined an oil is, the more likely it contains phospholipids and the valuable fat-soluble vitamins A and E. Soybeans and avocados are excellent sources of phospholipids.

When shopping for oils, choose unrefined and cold-pressed versions, which are the most nutritious. Avoid commercially processed oils as much as possible. Dyes, caustic solvents, stabilizers, preservatives, heat, and oxidizers are used to extract and prepare them. Avoid "cold-processed" oils, which can involve the use of chemical solvents if not heat. Remember that high heat turns even the highest-quality oils into hard-to-digest, denatured foods with carcinogenic by-products, and such a toxic concoction is sure to irritate the intestinal walls and interfere with good digestion.

There are other reasons to be concerned about specific vegetable oils that are not considered healthy. Palm kernel oil is a naturally hydrogenated vegetable oil used widely in confections because it creates a thick, creamy texture. Unfortunately, it's not easy to digest. Use of safflower oil is discouraged by practitioners of Ayurvedic medicine, who claim it interrupts the assimilation of calcium and creates gallstones. In addition, safflower is a heavily sprayed commercial crop and, like cottonseed, is not regulated by the Food and Drug Administration since, like cotton, safflower is not a food. Cottonseed oil is the most common ingredient in cheap vegetable oils, and cotton is typically treated with more pesticides than food crops.

The important point for food combining is that oil depresses appetite, inhibits stomach motility, and delays gastric secretions. Creams, gravies, butters, and oils taken in the same mouthful as nuts, cheeses, eggs, or meat create a multifaceted and extremely complicated meal. The same is true for fat and starch combos. The digestion of French fries is very slow and difficult, for example, because the potato is impregnated with cooked oil, and the oil must be dealt with before starch digestion can begin.

Lemon and green vegetables combine very well with oils. Green vegetables, which are rich in chlorophyll, counteract the depressive effects of oils on the digestive process.

Other Issues That Influence Digestion

Water with Meals

When it comes to food combining, the issue of drinking water with meals stands out as one of the most controversial. It is alleged that water dilutes stomach acids, prolonging the time it takes for food to digest. And drinking too much water with a full stomach can act as a flush, forcing the stomach to empty its contents prematurely. But that's no reason to stop drinking water with *all* foods.

Water is a natural component of many foods. When you eat foods with a high water content, such as watermelon, drinking a modest amount of water at the same time is harmless. Similarly, having water with apples or peaches is not detrimental to their digestion, since these fruits are mostly water and move through the stomach quickly. But avocados and coconuts are examples of non-watery foods. And coconut is loaded with fiber, which stimulates the secretion of hydrochloric acid to break down the fiber. Limit water consumption with such foods.

Green leafy vegetables of all kinds, including green sprouts and salad greens, are 80 to 90 percent water. Again, drinking some water with these foods doesn't usually create a problem. Raw high-fiber vegetables, such as beets, cabbage, and carrots, require stomach acid to soften the fiber, which isn't digested (the cellulose in these foods acts primarily as roughage). Still, drinking water with these foods only mildly detracts from digestion. Starchy vegetables, such as broccoli, Brussels sprouts, and cauliflower, take on an even greater amount of water when steamed or cooked in water. It's also safe to drink some water with these foods, although not as much as you might drink with leafy greens.

Dried fruits are concentrated, high-fiber, low-moisture, high-sugar foods. They require some stomach acid to soften the fruit fiber. Drinking water can also be of value here. These fruits are so dry that the water softens them and acts as a lubricant and solvent. Better than drinking water with dried fruits is rehydrating them before eating. When this isn't practical, drinking water helps reconstitute these fruits in the stomach.

Starchy vegetables, such as a baked potato, also need lubrication. Ideally, this should be provided by saliva or by pairing the potato with foods that have a higher water content. For example, a salad eaten with the potato helps keep the stomach lubricated. A meal of just potatoes and bread, however, would be so dry that you would instinctively want to drink water. In this instance, sipping a judicious amount of water would keep the stomach muscles churning and move the food around. The key is allowing for normal motility of the stomach by either adding small amounts of water or mixing drier, starchier foods with lubricating foods, such as vegetables and salads. So, a bit of water with a dry, starchy meal can be helpful, but too much will dilute valuable stomach acid and enzymes.

More caution is required when it comes to protein, fats, and oils. When a lot of water is consumed with a protein meal, it dilutes the stomach's powerful hydrochloric acid, rennin, and pepsin. Drinking water with oil-rich foods, such as avocados, is also problematic. Water and oil don't mix. Avoid drinking water with proteins or oils because it will prolong the length of time needed for digestion.

Cold and Hot Drinks

Ice-cold drinks chill the stomach and slow down digestion by dropping the operating temperature of the stomach and slowing gastric secretions. When this occurs, food stays in the stomach longer, and extra energy is required to raise the stomach temperature back to normal. Hot drinks also shock the system, although to a lesser extent. Basically, the closer drinks are to normal stomach temperature, the less strain they put on the digestive process.

Food Allergies and Sensitivities

Food allergies and sensitivities can also affect digestion. If you have an allergy to, for example, milk, chocolate, strawberries, peanuts, or soy, it will be harder to digest these foods. Many people have trouble digesting cow's milk because they lack the enzyme lactase, which digests the sugar lactose in milk. As we grow older, we tend to produce less lactase, developing problems with dairy that were not present before. Some ethnic groups have an inherent lack of lactase, making dairy a problem food from day one. Soy milk is also high in protein and fat and can be difficult to digest simply because it's so complex.

Don't assume that all liquids are easy to digest. Everything is relative. Yes, soy milk is easier to digest than soybeans, and milk is more digestible than cheese. But if you have sensitivities to these items, they will be difficult for you in any form. Learn your limits. If you suspect a problem, test yourself by having only small amounts at a time. Try different brands, dilute liquids with water, or avoid problematic foods and liquids completely.

Food Combining: Nature and You

What about Nature? She creates many complex foods, such as peanuts, that combine protein and starch. So why must we be so careful with our combinations? Nature does create complex foods. But the stomach recognizes a peanut as a single food, digesting the starch first and then secreting enzymes to digest the protein. This is very different from managing a man-made combination that requires different digestion times and enzymes. A good example is a cookie. It's one thing for the stomach to deal with natural grains, but when we grind grains into flour and add sugar, nuts, chocolate chips, and more, we have a food that is several times more complex than just the original grain. From this, the stomach receives conflicting signals, and ultimately digestion suffers.

Okay, so we all eat less-than-ideal food combinations—even if we know better. What can we do about it? We can buy the brand of peanut butter without added sugar. Don't eat the fruit that is served with your salad. Push aside the orange juice that comes with your breakfast muffin. Choose the cookie that is made without nuts. And so on.

In other words, you can control the amount of clashing foods in any given meal—in both big and small ways. When you season your rice, use less oil. When you're at a party and there is a smorgasbord of many different foods, concentrate on the vegetables and starches, avoid the fruits, and only dabble in the protein dishes.

Even the worst combinations can be properly digested if eaten in small enough amounts. If you have a bite of someone's peanut butter sandwich on an empty stomach, for example, the negative impact on your stomach will be negligible. And if there is only a thin layer of peanut butter on the bread, the bread becomes the dominant food. The stomach digests the bread first and works on the peanut butter later. If there is a lot of peanut butter and a thin slice of bread, the stomach digests the peanut butter first and the bread is finished later. But if that sandwich has a lot of jam, a lot of peanut butter, and a lot of bread, it's entirely another matter. To the digestive system, such a meal is a bear, working your system hard and leaving you exhausted.

The toughest combinations (see box below) are starch and protein, sugar and protein, fat and protein, and multiple types of different proteins, such as cheese and nuts. These combos all require the production of a lot of stomach acid and long digestion times. Combinations involving sugars and starches are not as burdensome because the digestive challenge is not as extreme. Both of these depend relatively little on the stomach for their digestion. If you eat a bad combination with a fruit, the stress on the system is much less than if you eat a bad combination with a steak.

The Four Toughest Food Combinations
- protein and starch
- protein and sugar
- protein and fat
- various proteins combined

A Day of Perfect Meals

This is an ideal day—a day of perfect food combining! Start off with the easiest of all foods to digest—water. You can't get into trouble with water, unless it's polluted! Drinking a full glass (between 16 and 32 ounces / 500 milliliters and 1 liter) or more of pure water is the best way to start your day. It flushes out your stomach and gives you a clean start.

Pre-Breakfast Drink

Next comes what could be your most nutritious meal of the day—a fresh vegetable or fruit juice. Get out your juicer. Choose veggies according to what's in season: beets, carrots, kale, parsley, spinach, or the always seasonal alfalfa sprouts. Or enjoy a fresh fruit juice made from apples, oranges, grapefruits, or grapes. You'll be amazed at how much better freshly made juices taste compared to the bottled variety. Allow at least fifteen to twenty minutes for the juice to leave the stomach before introducing solid food.

Breakfast

Good morning! Today I'll be serving brown rice cereal sweetened with rice malt. (Alternatively, try any grain cereal, such as oatmeal or grits.) Rice malt is maltose, a disaccharide sugar derived from rice. It's only mildly sweet and, if any sugar is going to be compatible with rice cereal, it's rice syrup. If you chew very well and thoroughly mix the cereal with your saliva, you can minimize the inhibiting effect that the sweet malt has on the secretion of the enzyme ptyalin. Want to add raisins or bananas? Yes, they're delicious, but the more sweets you add, the more you compromise the digestion of the starchy rice. But if you feel up to it, add just a small amount.

Lunch

Now comes the most traditional of all lunch foods—the sandwich. First choose the best bread you can find, preferably made from stone-ground, organic whole grains with no white flour. (If you're allergic to wheat, choose rice bread or any other gluten-free bread.) Next, add sprouts or salad greens, mustard, tomato, pickle, mayonnaise, and potato chips on the side . . . RING! RING! It's the food combining alarm! . . . cautioning you that this conventional sandwich is a recipe for digestive disaster!

To improve digestion, limit the amount of tomato and hold the pickle and mayo. Acidic foods, such as tomatoes and pickles, interfere with the digestion of starches, such as bread. Make a compromise. Since tomato is only mildly acidic, add one slice, but put back that pickle! Pickles are cured in vinegar, a very strong acid. Mayonnaise is a protein that contains vinegar along with saturated oil and sometimes eggs—and it combines poorly with many other sandwich ingredients. If you don't want to give it up, smear on only a thin layer.

Now for the potato chips. Isn't one starch at a meal enough? Okay, more than one starch is acceptable, since starches are not that different or complex. But why must it be potato chips? Chips are deep-fried in oil and are largely indigestible because the oil has permeated the potato thoroughly, coating all the starch and prohibiting starch digestion. So nix the potato chips and any other fried foods. Alternatively, choose baked potato chips or corn chips or, even better, slice up potatoes and bake your own chips.

Before-Dinner Snack

Keep it simple. Have a piece of fruit, a hot drink, or a smoothie. If you enjoy herbal tea, choose one that boosts digestion. Cinnamon, ginger, and peppermint are all wonderful digestive stimulants to clear the stomach and prepare it for the next meal.

Herbs that Stimulate Digestion

- cardamom
- cinnamon
- dandelion
- ginger
- peppermint

Dinner

This evening's menu starts off with a glass of fresh fruit or vegetable juice to cleanse the palate. Next is a salad of fresh greens and vegetables in season, which should precede heavier foods. The vegetarian main course features cubed tofu sautéed in olive oil, tamari, and a touch of dark sesame oil, with freshly grated ginger, garlic, and sautéed snow peas, green bell peppers, and mung bean sprouts. On the side is a bowl of long-grain brown rice.

What a magnificent combination! A vegetable dish with one protein—tofu. Yes, it's cooked with oils, and they complicate a meal. But olive oil is one of the most digestible oils and holds up well under cooking because of its moderate smoke point. A dash of dark sesame oil provides extra flavor. Ginger stimulates digestion in addition to adding its distinctive flavor. The vegetables, with their various textures and nutrient contributions, all stand up well under light cooking.

Just Desserts

Now it's time for something sweet. One hour or more after finishing the main course, enjoy a modest dessert. Most desserts are complicated because they usually involve flour, dairy, and a sweetener. The sweetener slows the digestion of the flour, and the dairy slows the digestion of everything. If you pick milk and cookies, you're mixing dairy, a starch, and a sugar. If you pick lemon-tofu pie, you have wheat in the crust (starch) and tofu (protein), a sweetener, and an acidic fruit (lemon) in the filling. You would be making a superior food-combining decision if you were to choose fresh or dried fruit instead, served alongside a hot cup of tea. However, if you prefer cookies or pie, have only one or two cookies or a small slice of pie. You can handle difficult combinations as long as they're in manageable amounts. Remember, the bigger the meal, the fewer enzymes are available to digest dessert.

The Results of Poor Digestion

Our discussion of food combining has focused mainly on the stomach. When the stomach isn't able to do its job efficiently, there are repercussions, such as heartburn. And as is the case in any assembly-line process, what happens early on affects everything down the line. During the process of digestion, this means the intestines will take a hit, resulting in flatulence, imbalance, and disease. In fact, you may have heard the expression "the source of all disease begins in the colon." The colon is part of the large intestine, and good colon health is fundamental to good health.

Heartburn

Chronic heartburn—that burning feeling in the center of the chest—is also called gastroesophageal reflux disease, often referred to as GERD or just "reflux." Reflux pain in the chest can be so severe, it's frequently mistaken for a heart attack! When GERD sufferers want relief, they usually reach for Tums, Maalox, Alka-Seltzer, and similar popular over-the-counter medicines. These are some of the best-selling drugs in the world! Unfortunately, they contain calcium carbonate (chalk), magnesium, and aluminum hydroxide that can create dependencies and have side effects. An effective, safe, and affordable home remedy uses baking soda to neutralize excess acid. Just mix a teaspoon in a glass of warm water and drink it at the first sign of heartburn.

Natural Treatments for Heartburn

- aloe vera juice
- baking soda
- cabbage juice
- chamomile tea
- cinnamon
- dill
- gamma oryzanol
- ginger tea
- goldenseal tincture
- L-glutamine supplements
- licorice
- potato juice
- slippery elm bark

Chronic heartburn is a warning to reduce stress, lose excess weight, and reformulate the diet. Limit consumption of foods and beverages known to trigger heartburn, such as alcoholic drinks, chocolate, citrus fruits, coffee, fried foods, high-fat dairy products, tea, tomatoes, and spicy foods.

In addition to eating the wrong foods and overeating, heartburn can also be caused by an enzymatic deficiency. Supplementing with enzymes may improve symptoms. Conventional antacid medicines can compound the problem because they inhibit the activity of hydrochloric acid and pepsin, thereby suppressing the digestion of protein.

Several herbs can help heartburn. Cinnamon, dill, ginger, and licorice all function to either stimulate digestion or reduce inflammation. Slippery elm bark, available as lozenges or tea, soothes the irritated and inflamed lining of the stomach and digestive tract, as does aloe vera juice. Ginger is a proven remedy for not only acid indigestion but also flatulence and nausea. Drink hot ginger tea or add fresh ginger to carrot juice. Goldenseal, available as extract or tincture, is a tonic and astringent for the mucous membrane lining of the gastrointestinal tract. It helps heal inflamed membranes and soaks up excess stomach acid. Licorice, especially deglycyrrhizinated licorice, has a long herbal tradition with scientific backing for treating colic and gastric ulcers due to its anti-inflammatory properties.

Raw, fresh cabbage juice is very soothing to the stomach and can even treat ulcers. Raw potato juice, including the skin, can help heal the stomach and lining of the esophagus, reducing the effects of heartburn. These vegetables can be juiced with carrots and consumed regularly.

Supplements also can help. Magnesium glycinate is a highly absorbable magnesium chelate that is used as a gastric antacid for sensitive individuals. Gamma oryzanol, a component of rice bran oil, alleviates heartburn along with gastritis, nausea, and abdominal pain. L-glutamine is the most important amino acid for the growth and repair of intestinal tissue. Supplements are available as capsules or powder.

Common Gas-Producing Foods

- beans
- cabbage family vegetables
- chocolate
- dairy cheese (hard) and milk
- dried fruit
- onions
- sweets
- wheat

Flatulence

Long-term solutions to flatulence are dependent upon diet but are also aided by exercise, supplementation, and stress management. When it comes to diet, beans have acquired the stigma of being flatulence-causing foods. Beans are not the only foods that cause gas, however. Milk and milk products, high-fiber foods, allergenic foods, and imbalances in the intestinal flora can all cause gas, or flatus.

One reason that beans cause gas is the presence of oligosaccharides, which are carbohydrates that are hard for the digestive system to break down. Oligosaccharides are also found in grains, seeds, and the cabbage family of vegetables, such as broccoli, Brussels sprouts, cauliflower, collard greens, kale, kohlrabi, rutabagas, and turnips.

After these foods pass through the stomach, bacteria in the intestines complete the digestion; in the process, these bacteria produce gaseous by-products, such as carbon dioxide, hydrogen sulfide, sulfur dioxide, nitrogen, and methane, which contribute to flatus.

Soaking and rinsing beans and other foods containing oligosaccharides, such as grains, can help eliminate gas. Multiple soakings and frequent water changes are most effective. Sprouting beans also transforms the oligosaccharides. Fermented foods, such as sauerkraut, tempeh, tamari, and miso, create cultures of active bacteria that also split the oligosaccharide bonds and aid digestion.

In dairy products, milk sugar is the culprit that causes gas. The complex milk sugar lactose is too difficult for many people to digest. Undigested lactose often ends up in the colon, fermenting and generating flatulence. Cows' milk is, after all, meant for baby cows—not humans. Consuming hard cheese and other solid milk products increases the digestibility challenge. Remember that milk is often a "hidden" ingredient in other products, such as cakes, cookies, and puddings, which could also cause digestive problems.

Certain grains, such as wheat and oats, are also sometimes responsible for flatulence. Gluten, found in wheat, barley, and rye, can be a problem for those who are sensitive to it. For anyone, gluten contributes to bulk, and too much bulk stresses the intestines and can aggravate a flatulence problem.

Insufficient hydrochloric acid (HCL) is another cause of flatulence. Some individuals, especially those over the age of fifty, no longer secrete enough stomach acid to fully digest their meals. Large pieces of undigested protein and fiber travel into the small intestine and colon, where they ferment. Individuals with low HCL should eat smaller, more frequent meals and strictly follow the food combining laws in this book.

To naturally increase the production of HCL and helpful enzymes, do deep breathing exercises prior to a meal. Outside of mealtimes, aerobic exercises are the ultimate solution because they help circulate the blood and lymph, enhancing oxygen and nutrient delivery to the digestive organs. To increase digestive strength, do fifteen minutes of aerobics and follow with a period of relaxation, deep breathing, and a drink of water, in that order.

> ### Charcoal: The Cure for Gas
>
> The best short-term remedy for flatulence is charcoal. Charcoal tablets are effective, efficient, and nontoxic. Dosage can be two to six 600 milligram tablets. Start out with the smallest dose until you become familiar with charcoal's effects. In addition to absorbing gases, it can also absorb nutrients. So use it only when needed and on an empty stomach. Take it either in the morning or before bedtime. Avoid eating until one hour after taking charcoal tablets.
>
> Be aware that charcoal will blacken the stool. Don't be alarmed. Because of this harmless side effect, you can use charcoal tablets to determine the time it takes for food to enter and depart the body.

Candida and Leaky Gut

Candida albicans is the term for a group of toxic, yeast-like microorganisms that inhabit the mouth, throat, and intestines. They live in the intestinal tract all the time, doing us no harm, provided their numbers remain in balance with the also-present beneficial bacteria. When this natural flora in the intestines fails to control the candida yeast population, symptoms develop. After a long-term presence in the intestines, yeast can develop into fungi that root themselves into the intestinal walls. The wall then becomes porous, creating a leaky gut—a syndrome in which toxins from the yeast and putrid food particles enter the bloodstream and weaken the immune system. A majority of leaky gut victims acquire the condition this way.

Whatever its origin, leaky gut can contribute to many common health complaints, some of which aren't typically associated with digestive problems. Crohn's disease, colitis, and celiac disease have been linked with leaky gut, as have allergies, anemia, asthma, fatigue, fibromyalgia, lupus, rheumatoid arthritis, and skin complaints, such as eczema and psoriasis.

The insidious leaky gut syndrome compromises immunity in numerous ways since 60 percent of the body's antibodies are produced in the intestinal tract. A weakened immune system makes us even more sensitive and vulnerable, creating a vicious cycle. If you suspect you have candida, consult your naturopath and get a stool analysis. This test identifies the quantity and types of microbes in your intestines and shows how well you are digesting food. For anyone with digestive troubles, this test provides vital information that can help uncover serious intestinal disorders before they become too hard to manage.

Repairing a leaky gut involves multiple steps, starting with a detoxification program and cleansing. The next priority is to eliminate the yeast, which can be done by taking herbal antimicrobial formulas and eating a diet devoid of wheat, sugar, dairy, allergenic foods, fresh and dried fruit, food additives, active yeast, alcohol, anti-inflammatory drugs, and antibiotics. Finally, replenish friendly bacteria, including acidophilus and bifidobacterium, and supplement with plant-based digestive enzymes until digestive strength is restored.

Conclusion

"You are what you eat" is a popular expression that underscores the importance of choosing healthful foods. Indeed, what we eat is paramount to our well-being. But, it is *how we eat* that influences our day-to-day comfort, energy level, and chances for longevity and lifelong vigor.

For the best results, keep the five laws of digestion in mind when you eat: watch your food quantity and the frequency of in-between meals, strive for regular mealtimes, eat consciously, consume foods in a sensible sequence, and think about the issues of chemical compatibility discussed here. Shoot for "the perfect meal" as often as you can and you will fend off heartburn, flatulence, cramps, and other problems of poor digestion. A lot of what is covered in this book are common-sense practices that you can incorporate right away. These simple disciplines, such as consuming less, will improve nutrient delivery to all your organs and glands. Successful digestion means better absorption and assimilation, and that will keep you feeling balanced, strong, and full of energy. Eat well, live well, and you will thrive.

ABOUT THE AUTHOR

Steve Meyerowitz was christened "Sproutman" in the 1970s in a feature article in *Vegetarian Times* magazine because his New York City apartment was always filled with gardens of mini vegetables. They were part of his life-time fight against chronic allergies and asthma. After twenty years of disappointment with conventional medicine, he became symptom-free through his use of diet, juices, and fasting. In 1980 he founded The Sprout House, a no-cooking school in New York City, teaching the benefits of a living-foods diet.

Steve is a health crusader and the author of ten books, including *Power Juices, Super Drinks; Wheatgrass, Nature's Finest Medicine; Juice Fasting and Detoxification; Food Combining and Digestion*; and *The Organic Food Guide: How to Shop Smarter and Eat Healthier*. He has been featured on PBS, Home Shopping Network, and Food Network, and in *Better Nutrition, Prevention,* and *Organic Gardening* magazines. His sprouting inventions, such as the Hemp Sprout Bag, are sold nationwide. You can visit him at Sproutman.com.

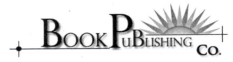

books that educate, inspire, and empower

A Holistic Approach to **ADHD** – *Deborah Merlin*

Weight Loss and Good Health with **APPLE CIDER VINEGAR** – *Cynthia Holzapfel*

Healthy and Beautiful with **COCONUT OIL** – *Cynthia Holzapfel and Laura Holzapfel*

The Weekend **DETOX** – *Jerry Lee Hutchens*

Understanding **GOUT** – *Warren Jefferson*

PALEO Smoothies – *Alan Roettinger*

Refreshing Fruit and Vegetable **SMOOTHIES** – *Robert Oser*

All titles in the **Live Healthy Now** series are only **$5.95!**

Interested in other health topics or healthy cookbooks?
See our complete line of titles at bookpubco.com or order
directly from:

Book Publishing Company
P.O. Box 99
Summertown, TN 38483
1-888-260-8458